TRANSFORM
YOURSELF
THROUGH
DISEASE

8 Steps to Reclaim
Your Health and Your Life

RORY REICH

TRANSFORM **YOURSELF** THROUGH DISEASE

8 Steps to Reclaim Your Health and Your Life

Copyright © 2019 Rory Reich

ISBN: 978-1-68309-241-4

Editing: Todd Hunter

Cover Design: Rory Reich

Author's photo courtesy of: Adam Crowley

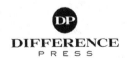

DP

DIFFERENCE
P R E S S

For my daughter, Sophia,

Thank you for your patience with me over the last few years, and thank you for showing me what unconditional love looks like. You have been the shining light, that I could always count on during my darkest times.

My love for you has no bounds.

TABLE OF CONTENTS

INTRODUCTION

I'm going to assume that you came across this book because you're struggling with a serious long-term health issue. Or, you're at the same place I was two years ago, when I allowed mine to get wildly out of control, and I was desperate to reclaim my health before it was too late.

I know those thoughts and feelings all too well. *Why is this happening to me! What did I do to deserve this?* I felt completely overwhelmed, lost, and scared. No matter how hard I tried, I couldn't seem to find the answers I needed to move forward. I was afraid I'd run out of time and I had no idea what to do next.

I'm here to tell you that there's hope. We live in a time where we understand more about the human body and mind than ever before. People all over the world are transforming their health and their lives on a daily basis. A healing crisis, and the journey it will take you on, is about more than just curing illness and disease. It's about deep introspection, profound learnings, and the opportunity for self-discovery that can transform you in unimaginable ways. It's a pathway that will provide you with the choice to get healthy, and to create a more meaningful life filled with passion and purpose!

The trick is, you must take charge of the situation and decide that you are in control of your life. That every choice you've made up until now has created the life you're currently experiencing. It's time to regain your power and to start taking the necessary steps to reclaim your health. This isn't going to be fixed by a pill, and it's not going to be easy. Real lasting change, will require you to change, while providing you with the opportunity to realize your full potential. So, get excited about creating a more empowered, healthy, and happy version of yourself.

What choice do you have? The universe is knocking on your door. You were delivered a wake-up call, and with that, an opportunity. The question is, what are you going to do with it?

My Story

*"Growth is painful. Change is painful.
But nothing is as painful
as staying stuck somewhere
you don't belong."*
– ANONYMOUS

I've been passionate about health and wellness for the last thirty years. During that time, I've been certified as a personal trainer, licensed massage practitioner, reiki master, certified sound healer, and transformational coach. I've also developed and launched multiple wellness-based businesses.

My passion started in my teens when I began training with weights. I quickly realized that through determination, hard work, and commitment you could rapidly transform yourself. I loved the feeling of looking in the mirror every day and seeing the positive changes that were happening to me. I became addicted! Over the next five years, I put on thirty pounds of muscle through consistent exercise and by radically changing my diet.

By the age of twenty-one, I was meditating and doing yoga for three hours a day. I had also given up drinking and become a strict vegan. My entire life revolved around the pursuit of physical and mental excellence. I had constructed what I thought was the ideal life, and was completely dedicated to studying and searching for truth in subjects like health, fitness, and spirituality. I was in my own little heaven, and this state of wellness, exploration, and discovery lasted until I was twenty-five.

Then one day, just like any other, I woke up, but I was completely exhausted. This was something I had never truly experienced. I had always felt great! I just assumed I had been putting in too many long hours at work. So, I decided to take a week off from all physical activity and give my body a rest. A week later, recharged, and excited, I went back to my favorite yoga class. It was intense as always, but I made it through to the end and I felt good.

Unfortunately, the next morning I awoke exhausted again. Frustrated, but assuming the best, I decided this time I would take an entire month off. Surely, I was just pushing myself too hard? I wasn't accustomed to doing anything halfway at that point in my life. But after a full month of rest and taking it easy, I went back to class, woke up the next morning and no difference, exhausted again.

I had no idea what was going on. I was living such a healthy life. How could I be feeling this way? Every action I took was dedicated to health and wellness. I was totally confused. I went to my doctor and he ran some tests, but everything came back normal. He didn't have any answers for me. So, I started trying everything under the sun, Eastern medicine, acupuncture, naturopathy, homeopathy, psychotherapy, energy work, cranial sacral, I even tried sweat lodges! If I thought it might make a difference, I'd try it. But no one had any answers for me. Everyone was just as stumped as I was.

It was a very difficult period in my life. Although I was still able to function and maintain a somewhat normal existence, my energy and vitality were drained. I had to completely manage everything I did just to keep myself from getting sick and rundown. Eventually, I stopped doing the things I loved, and the person I identified with was slowly fading away. No more books on wellness, no more meditation, no more yoga, and no more healthy lifestyle. I was complacent, and mostly just existing. Nothing I tried was working, and every time I'd get excited about a new potential solution, I'd end up being let down. Why bother?

Through all this, I was still able to hold down a job, and I eventually met my wife and started a family. From the outside, my life looked very ordinary and I was successful in most of my pursuits. But on the inside, I was only half there, and all along I knew something was missing. I thought it was just my health, which in a lot of ways it was. But more importantly, I'd lost was my passion for life. My desire to continue living. To live a life with purpose and to create something meaningful. I just didn't know what else to do.

Then one day it all caught up to me, and the life I tried so hard to keep in place finally came crumbling down. My wife and I had been having problems for a long time and had finally decided to get a divorce. I was still battling with my chronic health issues and I was working way too many hours at a job that I wasn't excited about.

I was feeling completely overwhelmed mentally, emotionally and physically. I was lost. Nothing in my life was working, and I kept thinking, is this it? Is this all there is to life? I didn't come here for this! I started questioning everything, including at that point, if I even wanted to continue living.

That was until I walked into my doctor's office to review my latest labs. As I entered, she said; "You look skinny, are you feeling ok?" I had progressively lost thirty pounds since I started having health issues, so being called skinny wasn't new to me. I told her I was feeling fine. I was just really stressed out and going through a lot personally.

That's when she proceeded to tell me, in the kindest way she could, that my latest test results indicated that I had a life-threatening disease. To say that my world was rocked would be an understatement. In all my years battling chronic illness, nothing had ever turned up on my labs, and I had never imagined I would hear those words. Shock doesn't do it justice. Me? Why me? How could this be? Are you kidding me? As if I don't have enough going on in my life!

She proceeded to tell me that I shouldn't worry, that I could overcome this. That I was the type of person who could do what was required if I could stay positive about the situation.

I really wasn't in the right headspace to hear anything else from her. I walked out of her office and never went back. Not because I was angry, and not because I didn't believe what she was telling me, but because no matter what I decided to do, Western Medicine wouldn't be a part of it. I think Western Medicine is great, if you're broken and you need to be put back together. But putting chemicals and pharmaceuticals into my body to bring it back to a state of balance goes against everything that I had come to believe.

If I had learned anything over the past twenty years, it's that Western Medicine was causing me more problems than providing solutions. I believe that our bodies and our planet provide everything we need for true healing. I was finally going to prove that to myself, and to everyone else if I had to.

But ultimately, I needed to hear this. There is no better motivation than the thought of death to turn your life around. I was tired of being sick and even more tired of getting my hopes up and not getting anywhere. I'd been living what felt like a half-life for far too long.

Twenty years! I was done! I was either going to find a way to get through this and come out a completely new person or leave this planet and everything else behind. This was my last chance. I had to take back control of my health and my life before it was too late!

Over the next two years, I began a journey of healing and a process of self-discovery. It ended up taking me around the globe to some of the most spiritual locations on the planet. I ended up forming a team of healers, mentors, and guides, who were finally able to get to the root of my health problems, and who nurtured and cared for me during this time. I came to realize that with chronic illness and disease, there is no silver bullet, there isn't just one issue or one cause, that led us to this state. It's multilayered and multifaceted, and this is why it can be so challenging to find the answers we seek.

It ultimately taught me that healing is a journey and that it's unique for everyone. True healing doesn't come in a bottle. A disease isn't just an inconvenience that we need to erase so we can get back to our regular lives. True healing doesn't just address your physical symptoms, it's a holistic approach that can transform your entire life.

It involves changing the way you eat, think, speak, feel, the company you keep, and most likely your entire set of beliefs. It's a message from your body, and the universe, that something is out of balance. And it's an opportunity to connect more deeply inside of yourself and change the trajectory of your life.

During this time period, I documented every conversation, every experience, and everything I learned. To be honest I wasn't sure why. It's just something I did. Eventually I began to realize that my story, my experiences, and my process of transformation may be of benefit to others. That this journey was potentially about more than just me. This has been my true desire for as long as I could remember, to help others and to make a difference. I finally realized that I had to truly help myself before that was possible. I eventually did. I have, and so I'm sharing what I've learned with you.

I'm happy to say that my health has been restored and that I feel like a completely different person than I was two years ago. I've never been happier and more excited about the future, and I have no idea where life is going to take me next. I love that! I see the magic in this world again and realize that as a species we are just beginning to truly understand our place on this planet, and the true power we all have over our health and our lives.

I know your journey will take you to new and uncharted places. I know it won't be easy. True change never is. I know at times, it will be really frightening, overwhelming, and lonely. But I can reassure you, that if you face it head on and use it as an opportunity and look for the learnings, then it can define you in ways that you could never predict.

I spent twenty years of my life on a healing journey. It was hard. It was mentally, physically, and emotionally draining. There were times I thought it would never end. It did. It ended when I decided to take back control, and to change my approach. To find others who had been through this, and to find the right help. As difficult as those years were, I'd never trade them in. I wouldn't have learned these truths, and I wouldn't be the person that I am today. And maybe, for the first time in a very long time, I'm happy about who that is.

I've spent over a decade developing processes of transformation for projects, teams, and people. All of them share the same basic attributes. During my healing journey, I created an eight-step personal process of transformation and I'd like to share it with you today. My hope is that it will help you reclaim your health and your life, as it did for me. So, what are those eight steps?

1. Healing Is a Journey

- It's time to get clear that illness and disease doesn't have to be a curse. But it is a wake-up call, and your process of healing and transformation is a journey. If you can embrace it, it's an opportunity where you can make radical changes that will redefine you in unimaginable ways.

2. Evaluate Your Life

- I consider this one of the most important steps of healing – getting to the root of the issue. You need to look at the entirety of your life, and not just the physical symptoms, if you want to create meaningful and lasting change.

3. Decide to Commit

- It's time to know why changing matters to you. What's going to keep you motivated on your journey of healing? What are the consequences if you fail? Are you ready to start taking responsibility for your actions so you can take back control of your life?

4. Take Back Control

- Taking back control of your life starts with taking back control of your thoughts, feelings, and beliefs. No matter how healthily you treat your body, a negative mind will eventually create a negative life. It's time to get in the driver's seat.

5. Choose Where to Start

- No worthy accomplishment happens by sitting on the sidelines. Here you'll learn to cast a wide net, get clear on some of your initial steps, and realize that you don't have to have every answer figured out, to just take the next step.

6. Just Take the Next Step

- With a clear direction in mind, it's time to start taking action. It's about taking the next step, even if you can't see the one right after that. Just continue to follow the clues and be open to altering your course when necessary.

7. Be the New You

- Here's where the hard work begins. It's time to start putting yourself and your healing journey first, no matter your situation. You must stop making excuses and prioritize your needs above everything else. Remember to focus on the positive aspects of your life and continually take steps in the right direction.

8. Practice Patience

- Real lasting change takes time, and this isn't a race. If you stay the course, every day you'll move closer to your goal. Remember to keep the end in sight, and to be patient.

My process is straightforward, and it worked for me. It breaks down each step into a set of guiding principles and as you work through this book, you'll see step-by-step, how it can help you too. If you follow this process, you will absolutely end up transforming yourself. The more you engage with it, the more natural it will become.

If we allow ourselves to embrace change, then health, happiness, and personal growth become a way of life. Resisting change is the easier course of action, but it only ends up costing us the sense of control and fulfillment we've been longing for. When you embrace change, you embrace life! Don't give up! Are you ready to get healthy and to live a more meaningful life filled with passion and purpose?

STEP 1

HEALING IS A JOURNEY

"Healing is a matter of time, but it is sometimes also a matter of opportunity."
– HIPPOCRATES

It's time to get clear that illness and disease doesn't have to be a curse. But it is a wake-up call, and your process of healing and transformation is a journey. If you can embrace it, it's an opportunity where you can make radical changes that will redefine you in unimaginable ways.

Change Takes Time

Real lasting change, and especially one that involves deep healing, takes time. It's not something that's going to happen overnight, and it requires us to get

to the heart of the situation to completely understand why we're here in the first place.

Often, we will point to an outside cause for
our predicament. Maybe another person, job, past
event, environmental factor, or a lack of something
we feel is crucial in our lives to make us complete.
But this is rarely the true cause of our problems.

Whatever brought you to this moment, it took
time. It didn't happen overnight, and changing
your circumstances isn't going to happen immediately. I know when we're frightened, we just want
the problem to go away, and we'll do whatever it
takes to get ourselves back to a safe place. One of
the most challenging lessons we must learn during
a health crisis is that it's a process, and processes
take time.

We Are Resilient

The human body is incredibly resilient. It can with-
stand an immense amount of neglect and abuse
over its lifetime. It can take years, and sometimes
even decades before signs of imbalance and disease
come to the surface of our lives.

Our bodies want to be in a state of complete health. It's their natural place of equilibrium. To be out of balance goes against the laws of nature, but we submit them to a tremendous number of daily stressors. Beginning with the unhealthy foods we consume. To the chemicals in the products we use. To the toxins we are subjected to in our environments, and to the daily mental and emotional stresses we encounter.

Eventually, these factors take a toll on our overall state of mind and our physical well-being. Sometimes we're aware of these factors, and the lifestyle choices we're making and their effects. At other times we're completely oblivious. Regardless, eventually they will catch up with all of us.

It's hard to say why some people are affected more, or differently than others. There are so many factors in our day to day lives that differentiate us. But all of us are influenced by our lifestyles, for better or for worse. Ultimately, we are all responsible for making the best choices we can in every moment to ensure we get the outcomes we desire.

Most of us know the choices we're making aren't always the best when it comes to our well-being. We aren't concerned as long as the doctor gives us a clean bill of health and we're able to maintain our desired daily routines. But even when we know our lifestyles aren't as healthy as they could be, it can be incredibly difficult to change them for the best. Why is this? Why do we make choices that go against our best interest? Why do we live lives that aren't in alignment with who we are and what we truly want?

I know from experience that it's sometimes easier to stay in a situation that isn't working and doesn't feel right, than to face the unknown and to make the choice to change our circumstances. Life can be confusing. It can feel overwhelming, and most of us crave a certain level of stability and predictability. Even if that situation isn't always serving us.

That is until we don't have a choice. That's when most of us realize our lifestyle choices and actions have brought us to a place where we are forced to change, or potentially stop living. I wish it weren't that way. I wish we all had the courage and determination to fully believe in ourselves, and to create the life we've always wanted. I know how real all those doubts and concerns can feel, and how paralyzing making decisions to change can be.

I believe some of us have just allowed our current experiences to become our new normal. We weren't always like that. There was a time when we were happy. When we believed in ourselves and the miracles of life, and we believed we could be and do anything we wanted. But somewhere along the way, we started to believe something else.

Somewhere along the way, we gained a new perspective. A perspective where we believed we were less than the people we compared ourselves to. We started to see ourselves in a distorted view, where we focused more on our shortcomings, and less on our unique strengths and passions.

If you're reading this book, at some point you probably felt that you've gotten off track. Your life isn't a reflection of your desires. You aren't fulfilled in one, or many areas of your life, and now you need to start taking back control of your life before it's too late. I know how that feels. I was there, and this is where I began.

Disease Is a Symptom

A disease is simply a state of imbalance. It's our bodies' way of telling us that we are out of alignment with our deepest desires, and that the lifestyle choices we're making are not in our best interest.

Getting out of balance is a slow process and has probably been happening under the surface for a very long time. Our bodies can only take so much, and when a disease finally surfaces, it's a wake-up call! It's our bodies' way of saying enough is enough, you need to listen to me.

But in our modern society, we don't really want to listen to our bodies. We're used to abusing them, oftentimes without noticeable repercussions. When we are forced to listen, it's an annoyance or inconvenience. We'd prefer to quickly deal with the situation so we can get back to our regular programming. We are a pill-first society who continually take drugs to mask our symptoms, without actually curing the underlying cause. Drugs work, and they can buy you time if you need it, but drugs don't cure.

Most medications are no more effective than a placebo, come with inherent side effects, and inevitably never cure the initial symptoms or disease. It has been shown that modern medicine is ineffective in curing 90% of acute illnesses.

If you have high blood pressure, is taking medication curing you? No, it's just masking the problem and potentially allowing new ones to manifest. Disease comes from our mental, emotional, and physical lifestyle choices. They are a reflection of our inner worlds. To get rid of disease, you must truly get rid of the cause. Which means you must change yourself, to change your physiology.

Our bodies never lie to us. They have an innate intelligence. They want to be healthy, they know how to heal, and if you listen, they will tell you everything you need to know. I definitely had not been listening to my body. I was numbing it with food and alcohol. I was tuning out on television every night, and I was overworking myself to take my mind off the fact that I was unhappy.

I just didn't know how to fix my situation. It seems so obvious now, and in some ways, so simple. We are all just so afraid of making the hard choices. Of demanding what we want in life and what we rightly deserve for ourselves. Our emotional connection to our circumstances can make it extremely challenging to see things clearly. For our bodies, the only thing standing in their way is us. There are no short cuts or quick fixes here. Real healing is a journey, and there is no express route.

Healing Is a Journey

Just like it takes time for a disease to manifest in our bodies and in our lives, it takes time for us to truly heal. Healing is a journey and there is no one right path for everyone. It's an individual experience that provides us with an opportunity for learning and growth. It's a holistic process that will challenge you to confront every part of your life, and that's exactly why it's happening. It's an opportunity to change your perspective on life and your situation. It's about deepening your spiritual connection, and it's about getting more in touch with your physical, mental, and emotional self.

You can fight this process, and you can try and resist it. But you've probably already been doing that for a very long time, and where has that gotten you? In all honesty, the last few years on this journey have been some of the most rewarding years of my life. I'm not going to lie and say it was easy, it wasn't! I've never experienced such intense moments of fear, sadness, anxiety, and self-doubt like that ever before. There were times when I was too weak to walk up a single flight of stairs. When I would sit alone in my house in tears, feeling inexplicably alone. When I was afraid, of whether I was going to live or die, and when I was confronted with important decisions regarding my health that just felt too overwhelming to make.

It took me a long time to find my bearings. But there was a turning point, where something changed inside me. Where I began to see the light at the end of the tunnel, and after that, I began to see and appreciate the experience for the opportunity that it was.

My words will never truly express to you the joy I encountered during this time. I would frequently shed tears in amazement, or in complete awe and with utter humility to something deeper and greater than myself. I couldn't have predicted any of this. I was so focused on my problems, that I wasn't even capable of imaging what was about to unfold.

The good news is that you don't have to. You just have to decide to change your perspective at this moment. To make the choice to see this experience as an opportunity for you to redefine yourself in every conceivable way. It's completely possible, and if you take it seriously, totally probable.

It's Time to Be Honest

Whatever brought you to this place, it's time to start getting really honest with yourself. It's time to start peeling away the layers until you can get to the core of the issues that have caused you to get off track.

You may be saying, "I just have a health problem. It's not my fault, the rest of my life is completely fine." But from everything I've learned over half a lifetime of studying health and wellness is that our physical bodies are just a reflection of our inner mental and emotional worlds. When we are truly happy, inspired, and living a life filled with passion and purpose, physical illness and disease are usually kept at bay.

Not to say this never happens, it does. Our environment has a huge effect on us as well. But most of us are wildly out of balance in terms of our emotional lives, our thinking, the way we deal with stress, and the treatment of our physical bodies.

STEP 2

EVALUATE YOUR LIFE

*"Ask yourself what is really important
and then have the courage to build
your life around your answer."* –
ANONYMOUS

I consider this one of the most important steps of healing – getting to the
root of the issue. You need to look at
the entirety of your life, and not just the
physical symptoms, if you want to create
meaningful and lasting change.

In this chapter, I'm going to challenge you to take a
step back and evaluate the entirety of your life, and
not just your physical symptoms. I want you to be
deeply honest with yourself during this process,
in the hopes that you will come out with a more

informed perspective on your life and the choices and decisions that brought you here.

Evaluate Your Life

Most of us spend some amount of time evaluating our lives but seeing the truth of our situations isn't always easy. I spent a lot of my time focused on what I didn't like about my life, but not knowing what to do about it, or even where to begin.

When my doctor gave me the news, it forced me to pull my head out of the sand and survey my life in a truly honest way. When I did, I didn't like what I saw. There wasn't a single area of my life where I felt successful or fulfilled, and in some areas, it was pretty toxic.

My marriage was extremely unhealthy and had gotten to an all new low. We had decided to get a divorce and were more or less living separate lives. I was unfulfilled at my job and felt unappreciated and misunderstood. My chronic illness was still unresolved, and I'd all but given up on trying to find a solution. The responsibilities of being a father and taking care of someone else when I was exhausted all the time felt totally overwhelming. I'd also completely lost my spiritual connection, which used to be my passion and purpose for existing. What had once been the centerpiece of my life was now completely non-existent. On top of all of that, my health had now taken a serious turn for the worse.

When I looked at my life, I wasn't following any of my passions or spending time on activities that gave me joy. I was just going throughout my day, from task to task, checking off boxes of responsibility and deriving almost no real excitement from any of it. I was just existing.

Now hopefully your life looks a lot better than mine did. But my point is, that almost every area of my life was out of alignment with my true wishes and desires. I was under so much stress and emotional turmoil that it's no wonder my body responded in the way that it did.

So, what did I do? I sat down, grabbed a pen and some paper, and started honestly evaluating my life. Now there are lots of ways to do this, but for the context of this book, I'll keep it simple (you can also visit my website for more in-depth questionnaires that you can print out).

There are six major areas of our lives. They are:

- Relationships
- Career
- Financial
- Health
- Passion & Purpose
- Spiritual

The importance placed per area will differ from individual to individual. But if you can maintain some focus in all areas, you will be more likely to achieve a healthy life balance. By focusing on each area of importance, we create awareness within us of what aspects of our lives need to be improved.

Relationships

This life area includes all your relationships, not just your intimate partnership. It's about your relationship with your spouse, your kids, your friends and with your extended family. All of these relationships have a huge impact on our time, health, and overall state of well-being. This is about deciding how much of that time, and what type of activities are important to you. Do you want to invest it in your kid's baseball practice, or do you want to spend time with your extended family on vacation? How about getting together with your friends after work? Regardless of the relationship type, this area is about connecting with the important people in your life.

Career

This life area is about your job or personal business. It might be an area you're really excited about. Maybe you've always known what you've wanted to do, followed your passions, and landed your dream job right out of school. Or maybe you've been in the same job for a long time, and although it used to be interesting and challenging, you now find yourself bored and wanting to try out something new. Our career is one of the most important areas of our lives. We spend an incredible amount of time here. If you don't have a job you love, but it meets your financial needs and you're happy with that, that's ok too.

Financial

This life area is about your finances. Obviously, it's heavily connected to your career and your ability to generate an income, but it's also about where you choose to spend your money, and whether you're making enough to meet your needs. Are you able to buy the home that you want? What about taking vacations regularly? Or are you always stressed about money? Is it something that keeps you up at night? Without the right financial resources, we can feel trapped in our ability to make change in our lives or pursue hobbies and past times that can bring us joy.

Health

Without our health, it's difficult to enjoy, and sometime even actively participate in the other areas of our life. But even if you don't feel unhealthy, it's important to be honest about the way you treat your mind and your body. Are you taking care of yourself? Are you exercising regularly? How about getting enough sleep? If you're not currently putting any energy into this area, chances are, you'll be putting a significant amount into it later in your life. As with every life area, take this one seriously!

Passion and Purpose

This life area is about how you choose to spend your free time. What do you love to do for fun? Is it vacationing? Or spending more quality time with your best friends? Maybe it's about pursuing your passions, learning to play an instrument, or donating your time to charitable causes. This is about the unique interests that make you, you. Are you spending enough time in this area of your life? Without time for our passions and purpose, life begins to just feel like work.

Spiritual

This life area is about connecting with that deeper part of yourself. For some, it's called religion. For others, it's just a profound need to unite and be part of something greater. And for others, it's about making a significant contribution to the world while they're here. It's different for all of us. The important take away is to understand what it means for you, and if you're spending quality time here.

Now, just take a moment and find a quiet place. Instead of focusing on your problems, try to get in touch with that deeper part of yourself that you may have been neglecting, that part of you that wants to be heard, and complete the following exercises.

Exercise 1:

Take out some paper and list out the six life areas discussed above. Now, prioritize each area of your life by importance. One is the area you value most and six is the area of least importance. This can always change over time, but it's valuable to see where you place your priorities in life.

Exercise 2:

Now, from one to ten, rate your satisfaction in each area of your life, as it currently stands. One being low, and ten being outstanding.

We aren't going to achieve a ten in all areas of our lives. Maybe you'd be happy with a seven or eight in certain areas and less in others, and that's fine. The importance of this exercise is to clearly see what your ideal is, and where you currently are in relation to that.

Decide Where to Focus

Now that you've evaluated your life, it's time to decide what areas you want to focus on. I'm not suggesting that while you're going through some incredibly stressful health crisis, you should divert your attention and try to rebalance all your life areas at once. I'm suggesting that you notice which of these areas are the most out of balance, and ask yourself, if there is the potential that it may be contributing to your health issues.

I can tell you from first-hand experience that they were for me. My marriage was taking a tremendous toll on my health. I know it was challenging for both of us, and I have no doubt it was affecting my wife in her own way. For me, and with the way I was dealing with my emotions, it was one of the major factors that had been slowly degrading my health over a long period of time.

If I would have completely ignored this area, and not dealt with the fact that I was living in an unhealthy situation that was causing me daily distress, there is no way my health would've improved. This was one of those areas I had to deal with! Confronting it was a requirement to reclaiming my health and my happiness.

So, I'm asking you to spend some time looking over your list and your answers and decide which areas of your life have to change, and have to change now! I'm not insinuating that you get up tomorrow morning and make a rash decision, but I am encouraging you to start being honest with yourself and to start adding this area to your daily focus list.

Don't worry about creating a plan right now. This section is just about getting clear on your situation, how things are going, and what you feel needs to change to get your life back on track.

Realize What's Been Holding You Back

Now that you have a list of life areas. I'm going to ask you to give some thought to what's been holding you back from making a change up until this point. Maybe you didn't feel that you needed to. Maybe you felt like your life was fine. Maybe you knew things weren't great but haven't known what to do about it. Maybe this health crisis has awakened you to the fact that things are out of control.

I've been amazed at my own ability to get comfortably numb even when my life was totally out of balance. Sometimes what we know, even if it is pain and unhealthiness, we fear less than the unknown. For me, I just didn't know what to do. I was confused and felt totally overwhelmed by the state of my life. I'd allowed myself to get to a place where I didn't really know or trust who I was anymore. I used to feel so secure in my thoughts and the perception of events in my life, but somehow, I had lost all of that. When you lose trust in yourself, it's incredibly challenging to believe that you can make the necessary changes in your life. Why would you?

It's easy when you feel confident, when you believe that you can achieve anything. When you've done it before, and the road ahead is familiar and clear. But when life feels overwhelming, and when nothing seems to be going right, making a change can seem unachievable, or unrealistic at best. Of course, this isn't true. We can all make changes. Even when we're at our lowest point. Especially when we're at our lowest point, because we only have one direction to go, you know, up.

I'm going to ask you to look over each of your life areas, and write down a few sentences about why you think this area is in the state that it's in. Once you have that, I'm going to ask you what you think is keeping it in that place. What are the reasons you can't make a change? Be honest. Brutally honest. This isn't about beating yourself up. It's about getting clear on the barriers that are standing in your way from having what you want in life.

Exercise 1:

Take out your paper, look over each of your life areas, and write down a few sentences about why you think it's in the state that it's in.

Exercise 2:

Now, write down the reasons you haven't made a change in this area. What has been holding you back?

Take a Holistic Approach

Whatever course of action you choose to pursue to reclaim your health, for true long-lasting healing your approach needs to be a holistic one. You might be wondering what the difference is between the areas of your life you previously evaluated, and a holistic approach to healing.

While they are connected, the areas of your life are about how you structure your life. What you value, and how each area is going in relation to your desired outcome or goals. The success or failure in a certain area, or in all areas, can have dramatic effects on your overall health, happiness, and well-being. When we're talking about a holistic approach to healing, we're specifically talking about the different areas of you, your core being, not your life situation. This is the part of you that is always there, regardless of the location, people, event, or circumstances you find yourself in.

When I began my journey, I didn't set out with the intention of treating myself holistically. It just naturally and intuitively unfolded in this way for me. Each piece of information I came across, and each new person I went to see, opened a new door and I just decided to step through it. At some point, I became less and less concerned with my health, and more interested in what I was learning about myself, the world, and my daily experiences. This passion for knowledge and the joy of exploration fueled me into new and uncharted territory. So, let's discuss what a holistic approach is in more detail. Here is the dictionary definition:

ho·lis·tic – adjective: Characterized by the treatment of the whole person, taking into account mental and social factors, rather than just the symptoms of a disease.

Modern medicine is finally coming around to the concept that there is more at play than just physical symptoms when it comes to treating illness and disease. But a holistic approach isn't just about the physical body either, it's about every aspect that makes us human. Here are the four areas I explored and documented, and ultimately made concerted strides in healing on my journey over the last few years.

They are:

- Physical
- Emotional
- Mental
- Spiritual

Physical

This is about your physical body. Your anatomy, organs, muscles bones, and systems. To heal, our bodies require us to eliminate the introduction of new toxins, to radically change what we put into them through our diet, and to use herbs and supplements to account for deficiencies.

It also requires us to remove the stored toxins in our bodies, so they can do what they are meant to, be healthy, and fight off sickness and disease naturally. We need to remove any barriers standing in the way so our bodies can do their job.

In summation:

- Prevent the introduction of new toxins
- Remove existing toxins from the body
- Feed the body healing foods
- Assist healing with herbs and supplements

Emotional

This is about releasing stuck and stored emotional energy inside of our bodies. Emotions are just energy-in-motion, and they are supposed to move freely through us. Even, and especially, when they are highly charged and negative. When they get trapped, unexpressed and suppressed, they cause blockages in our energetic bodies, which inevitably cause issues with our physical bodies. This is the foundation of energy medicine modalities such as acupuncture, acupressure, reiki, sound healing, qigong and taichi to name a few. When our energy moves freely without any blockages, our bodies can maintain harmony and balance.

In summation:

- Introduce energy stimulating practices
- Clear stored emotional blockages utilizing energy medicine modalities (breathwork, reiki, sound healing, etc.)
- Learn hands-on self-healing practices

Mental

This is about removing stress and negative thought patterns from our lives. It's no secret that 95% of our thoughts are unconscious, and a large majority of these are based on fear, doubt, and worry.

Getting in touch with and taking charge of our thoughts and our minds can dramatically affect our physicality. There have been numerous documented studies based on radical remissions using just the power of the mind alone.

In summation:

- Take stock of your daily thoughts and feelings around your life
- Utilize a daily meditation practice
- Research and get training in the latest information around mind control

Spiritual

This is about our connection to our soul. Whether you believe in a higher power or some greater source of truth and knowledge in the universe, our relationship with spirit is our reason for existing.

It's about your connection to something more meaningful, and applying purpose to your actions. It's imperative that you create meaning to your journey and your life and have a strong reason for living.

In summation:

- Strengthen your spiritual connection
- Find meaning in your journey
- Know your reasons for living

My holistic approach covers all of these areas, and focusing on all four will radically improve the time it takes you to heal. It will help you get to the root of the issues that are causing disease and will provide you the opportunity to connect more deeply with yourself, and in all new ways.

There is no one exact holistic approach to healing. The important takeaway is that you should be looking at yourself and every area of your life holistically, if you want to make radical, lasting change.

Can you imagine trying to overcome disease with a broken heart? Do you think it's possible to heal your physical body when every thought and feeling you're experiencing is sending out chemicals to your body that signal you are in distress?

What about losing your spiritual connection or desire to live? Our bodies respond to everything we think and feel. The answer is no. You can throw all of the drugs you want at your body, but if you are living in a state of fear, if you are lonely with no connection in your life, and if you've lost your reason to continue on, you're not giving your body a fighting chance.

Find an Example

One of the most important things I did on my journey and I continue to do to this day, is to find examples of others that are living the life that I want.

I've met so many incredible people over the last few years, and each of them had already gone through a similar experience. This is why they had the compassion, wisdom, and skills to help me navigate these challenges.

In my twenty years before this, I hadn't encountered a single soul whom I could relate to, and definitely not someone who had already solved my problem. But it's a different time. People all over the world are transforming their lives and sharing their journeys and strategies for the betterment of mankind.

We are all in this together. Disease is becoming all too common these days. Nearly half (approximately 45%, or 133 million) of all Americans suffer from at least one chronic disease, and the number is growing.

That is a staggering number! What is wrong with the way we are living? This is not normal. It's the opposite of normal. Somehow, we've been living in this distorted reality and we are accepting it. It's completely unhealthy and totally out of alignment with who we are and why we are here.

As a species, we need to make fundamental changes to how we're living, and how we're treating our planet if we're going to survive. I'm not trying to be doomsday; I'm just pointing out the fact that we can't continue forward like this. Things have to change, and they have to change soon. The good news is they are, and all of us have the opportunity to be part of that change.

I'm not asking you to change the world. I'm asking you to change yourself, and by doing this, you will indirectly be changing the world. That's how real lasting change is going to happen, one person at a time. So, don't focus on the problems of the world. Focus on yourself and become the change you want to see in the world. Become the example of a healthy, balanced, and happy human being. That's enough. That will create ripples in the pond that will inevitably affect others, and so on, and so on.

This doesn't mean you should turn your back on the rest of the world. It just means you need to get your life in balance first, so you can have the strength, confidence, and resources to take on even larger challenges.

I'm going to recommend that you start looking around your community. Start looking online, reading books, asking friends or colleagues, and start to find an example to model yourself after. Who's already solved this problem? It doesn't have to be just one person. I had many. People that lived close to me that I worked with on a weekly basis. Even many more well-known public figures that influenced my thoughts and beliefs through their written or spoken word. Start to find your tribe. Not all of them. Just start somewhere. The rest will follow when the time is right.

DECIDE TO COMMIT

*"Unless commitment is made, there
are only promises and hopes,
but no plans."*
– PETER F. DRUCKER

It's time to know why changing matters to you. What's going to keep you motivated on your journey of healing? What are the consequences if you fail? Are you ready to start taking responsibility for your actions so you can take back control of your life?

Take Responsibility

No matter the state of your life, at some point, you must decide to take responsibility for your situation. I'm not saying that you are the cause of your illness, but I'm saying we all have a part to play in our life circumstances.

Be honest. Are you treating your body like a temple? Have you created a life devoid of mental and emotional stress? Are you exercising regularly? Are you involved in loving, supportive, relationships where you're able to completely and honestly express your emotional needs?

I get it, we live in a complex world where it takes an inordinate amount of effort and discipline to be healthy and happy. Should it be this hard? I don't think so. But we've all created this reality. We've allowed our food and environment to be polluted. We've allowed the introduction of chemicals into our products. We support a medical system that relies on pharmaceuticals that inherently cause side effects. We've chosen speed over quality, and we've continually chosen to contribute to the rat race.

This was never anyone's intention. But we can't deny that we've all co-created this world, and it's only going to change when we accept responsibility and do our part. What does this have to do with you and your health? Because the way we treat our bodies, and the way we construct our lives, is a direct reflection of the way we treat our world.

We don't believe these conscious or unconscious choices will affect us. When they do, we feel powerless to do anything about it. But that's not true. We are powerful.

You can decide to take responsibility for your situation and for the choices you've made that have led to this moment. You can decide to make a different choice. You can decide at this moment to live your life differently, but you must first start by taking responsibility for your current situation.

No one did this to you. The world didn't do this to you. This is the moment where you stop pointing the finger and take full accountability for the circumstances and your ability to directly affect the outcome.

You can decide the outcome. You can become the change you so desire. But it all starts with taking responsibility for your life and your situation. Do not hand your power and your fate over to someone else. You are the deciding factor. Only you can make the difference between success and failure. Only you have that power!

Decide to Commit

Now that you've decided to take responsibility for your life circumstances, it's time to get committed to changing them. When it comes to personal transformation, there are few things more important than commitment.

Commitment means, doing whatever it takes. There is no halfway in commitment. It requires a tremendous amount of self-discipline, and first and foremost a belief in ourselves that we can change. Genuine commitment requires courage, sacrifice, and unrelenting determination.

Without it, we often get sidetracked by the sheer number of conflicting responsibilities that show up in our daily lives. Or by the poor habits we've become accustomed to such as laziness, procrastination, or self-limiting beliefs. When we can become fully committed, attaining our goals becomes much easier, and our choices become clearer.

Changing isn't easy, and it requires a significant level of consistent effort and determination. Whatever your goal, you will most likely have to make sacrifices in another life area to make progress towards it.

During my journey, I had to become relentless about how I chose to spend my time. This doesn't mean I had to completely forego a social life, or give up everything I loved, but I had to prioritize the activities that would allow me to reclaim my health over all others.

Sometimes these choices are easy, like when you're not feeling well and doing anything besides lying in bed is out of the question. At other times, these decisions are much more difficult, and take a tremendous amount of focus and willpower to stay on track.

That's why it's so important to evaluate your life. If you don't understand your priorities, it can be incredibly challenging to know what sacrifices to make when these decisions present themselves. If you're able to maintain a clear vision in your mind of what you want and where you are heading, you will eventually achieve your goals. When we're committed to change, anything is possible.

Embrace the Journey

Change doesn't have to be unpleasant. Once you've committed, your job every day is to embrace the experience, and ideally to fall in love with it. Can you imagine loving your healing journey the way you love your favorite food? What about loving it as much as you love your favorite activity? It can get to this place, it's possible, and it can become an obsession. Your biggest obsession, and one that brings you tremendous joy. Sounds crazy, I know.

You have to start to look for the wonder inside of the experience. Maybe you enjoy learning and can get fascinated by the miracles of the human body and what it's capable of. Maybe the human mind excites you, and you expose yourself to the latest science in this field, around the power it has over our bodies and our lives. Maybe your spirituality is important to you, and this experience can bring you to new depths and understanding of God and the universe.

There is so much new information available around healing, it's incredible. I'll admit that it can also be overwhelming at times. But it's up to each and every one of us to take in this new information, to hold onto the parts that resonate with us and to release the parts that don't. As I've mentioned, we're unique, what's important is what works and feels right for you.

There is true magic in the process of healing. It's one of the great mysteries of life. It will force you to ask important questions about why we are here, where do we come from, what happens afterwards, and what you believe. There are very few experiences in our lives that will challenge us to ask these types of questions and with so much meaning.

You're at a crossroads. As always, in every moment there is a choice. You have the ability to choose how you see this experience and how you navigate it. There is only one real option. Take responsibility, be committed, and embrace this journey. The other option isn't really an option at all. It will only lead to resistance, which will only lead to negative thoughts and feelings of power-lessness. Healing can't happen from that place.

Find Your Motivations

There was a point in my journey where I was confronted with an important question, did I want to live or die? This is a real choice that many of us are faced with in our lifetimes. It might sound silly, who wouldn't want to choose life over death. But we all know that plenty of people choose to willingly end their lives daily, and depending on your life situation, dying might not seem so terrible.

It surprised me when the question was asked of me. It wasn't the question that surprised me, but the fact that I didn't have an answer. I was indifferent. It took me a good week to come back to one of my healers with an answer. If you haven't already guessed, my answer was yes. If I had chosen no, then it's very possible my state of mind could have made that a reality.

The point I'm trying to make, is that I had to come to that answer for myself, as we all do in situations like this. For most I'm sure it's an obvious yes! Others might be tired of the fight and daily struggle they've already endured, and long for a pain-free existence beyond this one. I had to dig deep. Not to find my motivation as much as to decide if I was ready for the fight that lay ahead. Did I have the energy? Did I have the mental fortitude? Could I handle a fulltime job, take care of my daughter and still find the strength to take on this new challenge?

I'll be transparent, if it wasn't for my daughter, I'm not sure what my answer would have been. Twenty years of not feeling well, feeling despondent about finding new answers, and having zero confidence in our medical system didn't fill me with hope. Luckily, I found mentors, guides, and examples that did.

So, I'm going to ask you. What's going to keep you motivated on this journey? Mine was thought of losing my daughter. Her shining light, the boundless love I have for her. There was no way I was going to leave her without a fight. What's yours? What is your reason? What's going to keep you going day after day when the future outcome seems unclear? When you're tired, exhausted, and depressed? Find it, and hold onto it, it's going to make all the difference!

Set Your Intention

Now that you've reviewed your life, are clear on the necessity of taking a holistic approach, and have decided to get committed, it's time to create a vision for your future. You might be thinking: my vision is to overcome this health crisis and get back to my life! But I'm going to challenge you to get really clear on where you want to be six months or a year from now. How will your life look different than it does today?

If you're going to reclaim your health and your life, it's probably going to look dramatically different than it does right now. I want you to have a clear image in your mind of what that life looks like. Hold onto that image during this process, and use it to fuel you toward your goals of creating a happier, healthier version of yourself.

The image doesn't need to be complicated, in reality, the simpler it is the better. It needs to be something that you can achieve in the next six to twelve months. I prefer to make intention statements about each area of my life and review them daily as a reminder to what I want, so I don't forget.

Example:

In the next 12 months, I will fully reclaim my health by radically changing my diet (Life Area – Health).

This is a broad statement and it's not supposed to be an action plan. It's a goal. A year is a significant amount of time and a lot can be done, especially with a holistic approach. So, here's a little tip. I create and revise my intention statements every six months. They are extremely helpful for reminding me of what I'm trying to accomplish. Life gets busy, and sometimes we forget, especially if we are trying to make a change in every area of our life at once.

A little secret. I rarely meet my long-term goals in the time I've allotted. That doesn't mean I've failed; it just means sometimes change takes longer than we expect. I've been surprised at how long it's taken me to get my physical body back into balance. But how would I know how long it takes? This is my first time doing it with real success. We create these expectations of ourselves and of our situations and judge the outcome when we never really had the proper expertise to accurately plan.

The point is, for most of our goals it's not a race. The important part is that we inevitably get there. That we are making daily, weekly, and monthly progress, and continue to feel inspired and motivated along the way. As you make progress, you will get better at predicting change in a given area. You can come back and refine your intention statements at any time.

So even if you don't plan on focusing on your entire life right now, and only want to focus on your health, or one or two other areas, take a moment and make a statement for each part of your life. If you only have the time, and physical, mental, and emotional resources to focus on your health, do that! But it can't hurt to create an all-encompassing vision for your life. To get clear on what's important to you. So, when those resources do free up, and they will, you can divert some of your energy into other areas.

Exercise:

Take out your paper and create an intention statement for each area of your life. Start by making a six-month statement for your desired focus areas. You can use this to create a plan later in this book.

TAKE BACK CONTROL

"Whatever you hold in your mind on a consistent basis, is exactly what you will experience in your life."
–TONY ROBBINS

Taking back control of your life starts with taking back control of your thoughts, feelings, and beliefs. No matter how healthily you treat your body, a negative mind will eventually create a negative life.

I spent half of my life in a condition that I would categorize as, not ideal. I just couldn't understand why this had happened to me. What did I do? What could I have done differently? I would go over and over the events in my life looking for clues. Trying to put the pieces together so I would know, once and for all what to do.

No one could give me answers, and no matter how hard I tried, I couldn't find them either. With this latest diagnosis, I had to figure it out! So, I set out on a mission to reclaim my health, but ended up on a journey of self-discovery that completely transformed the way I viewed healing and the world around me. The information in this chapter has radically changed my approach to life. It showed me the power our minds have over our daily lives, and our ability to empower ourselves to take on life's challenges.

Your Thoughts and Feelings Create Your Reality

One of the healers I was working with recommended a video by Dr. Bruce Lipton. That video completely changed the way I looked at life. The content suggested, or dare I say scientifically proved, that our thoughts and feelings are responsible for creating our personal reality. What I loved about Bruce, was his ability to take complex concepts and simplify them so anyone could understand them, using the language of science. Which in this day and age, for a large majority of the population, has become our accepted universal source of truth.

In its most simplistic form, the concept in the video and of this section is known as the placebo effect. I'm sure you've heard of it. It's when patients are given a sugar pill (or equivalent) instead of actual pharmaceutical medicine, and a large percentage of them get better. This has been tested and proven time and time again. What this boils down to is the fact that if you believe something will create a certain effect in your body, there is a really high chance that it will. Even if it's just a placebo, which in essence, is just your belief in an outcome.

So how far can you take this? Can you cure yourself of anything because you believe you can? Well people have and are doing it as we speak. So what's the trick? The trick is you must find a way to truly believe it. You must believe it without a doubt and with every fiber of your being. I'm not sure if that sounds easy or hard. But as you can imagine, when you are confused, desperate, and scared, changing your belief about something is no easy task.

This isn't a switch that you can just turn on and off. It's a complete change in the way you think, feel, and act. It requires you to become a different person. If you want to be healthy, you must think, feel, and act like a healthy person. Do you believe it's possible to behave like someone that is sick or unhealthy and become healthy?

Every thought and feeling we have has an effect on our bodies. Imagine feeling anxious and scared for weeks or years on end. How do you think your body will respond? Well a lot of us are feeling that way, living in a state of constant worry, fear, stress, and doubt. Even if it's just on a very subtle level, over time this can have dramatic cumulative effects.

Exercise:

Watch your thoughts, and write them down as you go throughout your day. Evaluate them after an entire week.

When I did this exercise, I was amazed at how negative my thoughts were. I'd spend hours every day thinking about the worst-case scenarios in every area of my life. My divorce, my health, and my work just to name a few. I was astounded. I was spending all my time worrying about "what could happen," instead of, what I "wanted to happen."

Of course, this is to be expected. I was going through some serious stuff! I had a right to be scared! I had a right to be worried! But as soon as I realized this, as soon as I could really wrap my head around this truth, it changed my life forever. How can you ever have the life that you want, when you're constantly imagining everything that could go wrong with the life that you have? You can't!

I wasn't focusing on what I wanted. I was focusing on my problems and trying desperately to find solutions. What if the solution is simple? Focus on something else. Focus on the life that you want, imagine that outcome, and feel it and live it before it happens. You'd be surprised at how powerful that is. What if the real problem is our continual focus on what we don't want?

Imagine training for a marathon. You buy your running clothes. You research a training program. You decide on a marathon in some exotic locale and select one that is far enough out to ensure you can get in competition condition. Then the entire time you're training, you focus on all the things that might go wrong.

That you might hurt yourself. That you might get so busy at work that you won't be able to put in the hours. That your child might get sick and you'll be thrown off your training program. That you aren't really a runner. Who are you to think you're capable of doing this anyway? How far do you think you'd get? To run a marathon, you need to play the part. You need to live, train, and believe that you can do it. And ultimately, with that mindset, you will. That's what successful people do. They play the part before it happens.

For me, it just came down to common sense. It's not about pretending, it's about choosing. It's about deciding once and for all to take control of your mind, which is incredibly powerful, and spending every second of your day focusing on the life you want to create. Getting excited about the possibilities, about the details, and about truly being alive.

I realized I could complain about my circumstances. I could spend all day worrying about the things I couldn't control, and I could feel sorry for myself. But none of this would do any good. It just made everything worse. The outcome of every area of my life hadn't been determined yet. But in my mind, I was already deciding that things weren't going to go my way. Not anymore! Don't they say hope is the best medicine?

Your Words Have Power

If your thoughts and feelings create your life, the words you use are just as critical. Everything you say to yourself, or someone else, carries tremendous power. Can you imagine telling a child that they're stupid, every day of their life? Sounds horrible doesn't it? But we do it to ourselves all the time. We are constantly talking about how tired we are, or how sick and tired we are of this situation or that person. How stupid we are for doing this or that. We often think and say incredibly unhealthy things to, and about ourselves. We are constantly limiting ourselves with the vocabulary we choose.

I hear this all the time. During my daily interactions and with the people I coach. If you really learn to watch your language, and the language of those around you, you'll be surprised at how dis-empowering it can be. It's just another example of how we really feel about ourselves and the world around us.

You might be laughing and thinking how trivial this sounds. But your words are programming you, and others. If you're constantly telling your partner about their shortcomings, do you think they'll improve or decline with that type of language? Is that how you'd talk to a child? Do you think it would encourage them to change?

Our language, when used accordingly, can encourage and uplift others. It can make them believe in themselves in a way that might not have been possible before. What if you used that same type of language on yourself? What would happen if you only said positive things to yourself every day, and for the rest of your life? Don't you think that would have an effect on you? It would, and it is!

I'm not talking about mantras or affirmations, although I think those are great! I'm talking about ceasing to say negative things about yourself, or anyone for that matter. Your voice is a weapon, you can use it for good, or you can use it to cause harm. Once again, it's your choice. It's one of our greatest superpowers.

Exercise:

Watch your words and the words of those around you for a week and write down your findings.

Your Beliefs Are Limiting You

After these realizations had sunk in, it felt like a huge milestone. I had become aware of a part of myself that I just hadn't truly seen before. Now, this was also because my situation had heightened my normal ways of *being* from a three to a ten. Everything felt exaggerated. This crisis had exposed parts of me that I had hidden away from the world, and from myself. But this was only part of the story. Somewhere in this process, I realized that my beliefs about myself were pretty unhealthy as well.

The journey I was going through was bringing everything to the surface, and I didn't like the person I had become. I had lost all my confidence, and felt like a shell of a man. Was I always this way?

Was I just hiding it from myself and from everyone else? It was so hard to get clear on what the truth was. My mental chatter and emotions were so intense that I was starting to lose track of reality. I couldn't tell if this was the real me, or just me in this extremely intense situation. I can tell you without a doubt that I was finally encountering parts of myself that had been buried very deep and for a very long time.

What I realized is that I had told myself stories my entire life. Some stories were positive, a lot of them were not. These stories about who I was, what I was capable of, what I liked, and even my personality, were not always the truth. We construct entire personas based on the feedback we get from the world and what others tell us. You might be thinking, well that makes sense. Shouldn't we react to the feedback we get and make educated decisions about how we show up in the world? I mean if I'm terrible at singing, then I'm terrible at singing, right? Wrong!

These beliefs aren't real. They are just a set of agreements we made with ourselves to keep us safe. To define boundaries that we can exist in that ideally meet our needs. Unless they don't. I realized I was full of limiting beliefs. But these beliefs were usually just a way to keep me protected and to keep me small. To avoid failure. To avoid looking foolish. To avoid not being perfect and to avoid being alone. I was trying incredibly hard to maintain a life of control. In doing so, I created a life where I could exist without taking a risk, but at the expense of knowing what I was truly capable of.

The only difference between you and the person who is living your ideal life, is time and a positive belief in themselves. No one who has ever accomplished anything meaningful did so by staying small. By not taking chances. By continually worrying about what others were thinking about them, and about whether they were doing it exactly right.

We are constantly telling ourselves what we can't do. I see it every day. We look around at others and are amazed at the lives they have created. Somehow, these superhumans were born different. They're special. That explains it. But in reality, somewhere along the line, they created a vision for their future that wasn't small, and they believed in themselves enough to keep going. No matter what!

It's time to get clear. You're capable of anything you set your mind to. There is absolutely no difference between any of us, outside of our thoughts and our beliefs. People have overcome tremendous odds to reinvent themselves and become living examples of what's possible. They didn't do it with money, or connections, or fame, they did it with heart and a belief that they could.

Exercise:

List out all your beliefs. Your positive beliefs in yourself and what you are good at, and your limiting beliefs about what you aren't good at, and what you can't do.

Your Life Is Happening for You, Not to You

I was told by several people during my journey that I had created my health issues, and that I was capable of changing my circumstances at any time. I now understand the motivation behind these comments, and I know that they meant well. They were just trying to impart some knowledge and wisdom for my benefit. It's just hard to hear these things, especially from someone that's never experienced what you're going through. Which at that time in my life, was no one.

My belief, after twenty years of being on this journey, is that your life is happening for you, not to you. What exactly does that mean? It means that instead of identifying with the "problem," and feeling like these circumstances have magically happened, you must take a step back and realize that everything in our lives is happening *for* us. Every situation provides the opportunity to learn, grow, and to further define ourselves in this lifetime.

How can chronic illness and disease be an opportunity? How can it not? I know. That used to make me so angry to hear those words. But I've now come to realize the truth in them. I've met so many people over the last few years who, like me, experienced an incredible crisis in their lives, only to come out the other side completely transformed.

I've realized that's why we're here. We're not here to avoid pain, or to surround ourselves with material possessions and sit on beaches for a hundred years. We're here to experience it all, we're here to learn, and we're here to grow. This doesn't mean we can't enjoy life to the fullest. It just means life is going to have its ups and downs. When you can accept this, you can realize that it's during these challenging times that we're growing the most. We're being forced to face head on many of the things that make us human. Loss, death, betrayal, heartbreak, failure, and rejection to name a few.

Have you ever gotten to a place in your life where you're so comfortable, but bored out of your mind? We long for this place of security and safety where all our needs are met, and we don't have to worry. But most of us are blessed with an incredible amount of comfort and health compared to people in some parts of the world. We cannot avoid discomfort. We can only change our mindset around it. We must see that it's part of life, and if we face it head on, it can be incredibly healing and beautiful.

Your Experiences Are Your Teachings

Our souls long to know everything, and that includes the challenges in life. We are spiritual beings in human bodies, and we came to this planet to experience. This isn't the first time and it certainly isn't the last. We came here to learn and to grow, and our experiences are our teachings. We can't avoid them, and deep down you don't want to. Salvation from misery and heartbreak, happens through embracing our fears and finding the courage to transform them.

Every situation in our life offers us an opportunity to redefine who we are. In every moment we have a choice, and by making that choice we are creating a new version of ourselves. That version is either in alignment with our goals and the direction we are consciously heading, or it isn't. In every encounter, and in every conversation, there is a message awaiting you. When you're clear on what you want, and you can hold it in your mind's eye, the universe will present you with clues.

Our task is to stay ever present to the information that's being given to us on a moment by moment basis. When you change your focus away from "why did this happen" to "what can I learn from this," you will remove your victim mentality and be able to see how you can benefit from the experience.

That doesn't mean you won't feel anything toward it. You should allow yourself to feel every experience fully. It just means you don't have to dwell on it incessantly. Feel it, look for the lesson, and choose the meaning and the story you tell about it.

CHOOSE WHERE TO START

"To accomplish great things, we must not only act, but also dream; not only plan, but also believe."
– ANATOLE FRANCE

No worthy accomplishment happens by sitting on the sidelines. Here you'll learn to cast a wide net, get clear on some of your initial steps, and realize that you don't have to have every answer figured out, to just take the next step.

Cast a Wide Net

Now that you're mentally prepared to start your healing journey, it's time to get a plan. Before you can do that, you need to get informed. I'll tell you from first-hand experience, there is a lot of information available on every health issue and healing modality you can think of. Oftentimes with conflicting viewpoints. This can be incredibly frustrating when you just want to get a clear answer.

Fortunately, and sometimes unfortunately, this is the day and age we live in. Where information is paramount but getting a concrete and agreed upon answer is often elusive. There are multiple reasons for this. There isn't always just one answer, or one way to get results. There are often many. And what works for one person doesn't always work for another. We are unique beings in many ways. The important thing is to set aside some time and just get started. I often find that the information I come across is exactly what I need at that moment, even if I don't realize it. It all just happens intuitively and organically.

Start with the internet, ask friends, and share your story with others. I'm always amazed how much information other people have to share with me that's valid for my experience when I allow myself to be honest and vulnerable. Remember, information and clues are everywhere and in every moment.

There is no perfect source of information. It's about casting a wide net, enjoying the process, getting informed and trying to see the magic of how answers can fall into your lap if you are open to receiving them in any form. I'm still amazed at the way I'm guided daily. Every single conversation, event, or piece of media I come across seems to be hand tailored for my experience. Sounds crazy right? Be mindful of this process, be curious, and pay attention!

Also, write everything down. I kept a journal of all my learnings and the information I considered important. I still constantly refer to it. It's a living document that changes as I progress. Mine is electronic because I like the flexibility of accessing it on any device and the ability to make edits and remove information that I no longer find relevant. I used it to write this book. I use it to remember important lessons, to stay motivated, and to remind myself of the progress I've made.

You Don't Need All of the Answers

This is important. Over the last few decades I've become an excellent planner through my work. I'm really good at it! I can see all the variables, and I know how long tasks will take. I can evaluate all the people involved, their strengths and limitations, and can create an action plan and schedule that will always get the job done on time and in budget.

It's an incredible skill to have, but it's not always necessary or helpful. When you're on a journey, one of self-discovery and healing, you can't accurately plan the route. There is no way to see all the pieces on the board, or how they'll come together and at what time. How could you possibly plan every detail around something as complex as the process of transforming your life? The answer is you can't.

The great news is you don't need to. The best thing you can possibly do for yourself is to just plan the next few steps, or even just the first step. Life and this process will unfold naturally, in their own time, and in a way you probably could never imagine.

The last few years have been an incredible adventure for me. When I started, like most people, I just wanted to fix the problem. I just wanted to reclaim my health so I could get back to my regular life. But as I've mentioned, my regular life was a mess and had completely fallen apart.

I totally misunderstood the opportunity the universe was providing me. It wasn't just about healing my physical body; it was about transforming every part of myself and allowing me to define a completely new vision of who I am and what I want in life. I didn't even see this at the time. So how could I have planned it? I couldn't. I wasn't supposed to.

Go with What Feels Right

When deciding where to start, you just have to go with the choice that feels right to you at that time. Which idea or direction gets you the most excited? Which one feels right in your gut? We intuitively know the right answers. But we are often too wrapped up in the mental chatter of our minds, or in the fear and worry around the outcome, to clearly listen to ourselves.

I know when I was in periods of immense fear and worry that I just wanted someone else to make the decision for me. I desperately wanted to give away my power and let someone more educated than me make the choice. Unfortunately, no one else can choose what's right for us. People will, when we put them in that position, but it's just their opinion, and completely removes the process of your inner knowing and intuition. Which is always right for you in every moment.

Over time if you can start to trust yourself and bring yourself to a point of stillness, you'll be able to ask important questions and be at peace with the process and answers that you come to. No matter what you decide you will almost always have the option to course correct.

Even in the worst extremes, you will get to a place that feels so wrong, that you won't be able to hide from the fact that you need to head in a different direction. The goal is to not let it get that far. But even if it does, remember, you've learned something along the way, you're stronger for it, and you have the power to make another choice.

There Is No Perfect Choice

Every day we're presented with the opportunity to make choices. Most are small, but oftentimes they feel really important. Instead of worrying about it, which is what I used to do all the time, I now just pick the direction that I'm most excited about and commit. This is the way the process should work. Research your options, decide what feels right, and then choose. No matter what I choose, there is always something of value for me in that experience. I always learn something new and continue down that path if I'm still excited about it.

It's the excitement that's important. It's about the feeling that what you're doing is right. It's not a mental process, it's an, energetic, emotional, and physical one. You are allowing yourself to be led by what feels right to you, not through some analytical process of the mind. It's not that the mind isn't important in making decisions, it's just that the mind cuts out your intuition. Your intuitive process is a feeling, a deep knowing, and it feels good when you're on the right path, and it feels bad when you aren't.

Intuition isn't some strange metaphysical concept. It's a natural part of being human. We all have it; it just isn't valued or recognized in our culture. It's another sense that can be developed and used like any other. It's like a muscle, the more you pay attention to it, the stronger it gets. All of us have had intuitive experiences. We just don't think about them when they happen, and that's the point. When you've had them you probably weren't thinking, which is what allowed it to work. It's about getting out of our minds and getting into the experience. It's about becoming a participant in the flow of life.

After you've researched your options, it's time to get started. Remember that there is no perfect choice. There are many paths we can take in life. Many paths that will bring happiness, success, and healing to us. There is only the choice you make at that moment. You almost always have the luxury of making a different choice if that one isn't working for you. This happens all the time and is part of learning and growing. The choice you make at that moment will lead you to the next opportunity and the next piece of information.

You must completely change the way you think about decision making. We put so much pressure on ourselves to make the right decisions in life. Somehow, it's been ingrained in us that there is always a right choice to be made. Where did that come from? Even when we feel our lives have gotten off track and we attribute it to the wrong decision we made in the past, that's not always accurate.

We fantasize that life is supposed to be a smooth ride. But no one's life is like that, and it's not supposed to be. When you feel like you've gotten off track, it's an opportunity to reflect, learn, and change course. That's it. Self-punishment, blaming others, and dwelling on it as a mistake have absolutely zero benefits.

What did I learn, and what is my next choice going to be? Those inevitably are the only real questions to be asking yourself in every moment and every time you need to make a decision.

Don't Go It Alone

I didn't set out on my journey looking for mentors. I was just trying to get information and following the recommendations from people whose opinions I valued. With that said, I ended up creating a team who guided me during this time of transition and healing.

I honestly can't imagine how I would have done it without them. There are people in this world that have already been through a healing crisis. That have already learned these lessons. Who have so much wisdom, compassion, and knowledge that *we* just can't possibly possess when we start out. And that's exactly what this journey is all about. All of us, have the opportunity to take what we've learned and to help others. That doesn't mean it has to become your occupation, but you will inevitably help someone else with the information you gather along the way. We are all here to help elevate the human race. To raise the collective consciousness and to heal ourselves and the planet.

Every journey is unique. Every one of us has a new piece of the puzzle to offer up to humanity.

Medicine and healing are an art that in no way has come close to being mastered. We are all creating this masterpiece together. What part will you contribute? Just participating is enough. Just changing the way you think, just believing in yourself, and just being an example of a different, more conscious way to live, is enough. It's plenty!

You don't have to search out and find a mentor right away. I found my mentors organically through the process. I just realized I needed more of what these people had to offer in my life and on my journey. Having someone that truly understands what you're going through is invaluable. It's so difficult to do this alone. For twenty years I'd felt that way: alone! When no one could tell me what was wrong, or what to do to change my circumstances. When I wasn't meeting others that could relate to my experience, that was extremely lonely and hard. I wouldn't wish that upon anyone.

As I said earlier, the world is a different place now. There are many more people experiencing mystery illnesses and going through healing journeys. There is a wealth of information available and so many people to lean on. It's a different time.

I'm incredibly grateful for that. You can start your process by researching and finding someone who's already traversed this. You might end up with more than one, and you may transition between people as you go, and that's ok. Just remember to go with what feels right, and don't over analyze it. Don't get stuck in your head worrying about whether you're making the right decision. Get quiet, get clear, decide, and just take the next step.

JUST TAKE THE NEXT STEP

"Success is not final, failure is not fatal;
it is the courage to continue
that counts."
– WINSTON S CHURCHILL

With a clear direction in mind, it's time to start taking action. It's about taking the next step, even if you can't see the one right after that. Just continue to follow the clues and be open to altering your course when necessary.

Just Take the Next Step

Now that you've made a decision, it's time to get started. Remember, this doesn't have to be the perfect decision, you just have to start somewhere.

My journey took me in many different directions. The people and places I started with were not always where I ended up. But each person, and each event, taught me something that I used to propel myself forward and to continue down the path. I recommend starting small. Pick one thing to try, one person to meet, and just go for it. No matter what happens, you will leave with more information than when you arrived.

I still consistently search out and try new people and experiences. I spent my first six months researching and trying out as many things as I could. I did energy healing, breathwork, sound healing, naturopathy, homeopathy, qigong, and Chinese medicine to name a few.

Some of those I stuck with because they resonated with me, and the ones that didn't I just left behind. This is an opportunity for you to form your team and to explore you! Recommendations are great, and you should follow them if it feels right. But what works for someone else may not work for you. Just keep that in mind. It's your journey. You're the expert!

Continue to Follow the Clues

After you take the initial step, you just need to continue to follow the breadcrumbs. As I mentioned before, it's not always possible to have a concrete plan in life. I've found that most times in my business and personal endeavors, it works best when I release the need to control everything and just go with the flow. Following the breadcrumbs means looking for clues on what direction to go next, instead of trying to force a situation or have an airtight plan.

This can come in many forms and still happens to me daily. The key is to maintain a clear goal in your mind at all times. To keep your eye on the prize. When you know what you want and what direction you're heading, life will consistently bring you the necessary information to continue forward.

Each practitioner I worked with supplied a new piece to the puzzle, but they weren't necessarily a final destination. I'd often ask them who their favorite healers were in the city. This would inevitably lead me to three or four other incredible practitioners who I would immediately try out.

I'd do the same thing with each new person I met, until eventually, I found the team that worked for me. Where I felt safe. Where I felt understood, and where the experiences I was having were validation that I was on the right path.

Be on the lookout for breadcrumbs, they come in all different forms. Pay attention to the most trivial conversations and media that come your way and continue to share your story with others. I'm an extremely private person. Although you might not think that since I decided to share my experiences in this book. But I am. I didn't tell very many people over the last few years about what I was going through. It just wasn't a natural or easy thing for me to do.

Most of us don't want to burden others with our problems or be a complainer. I can see from where I'm standing now that every person is a potential breadcrumb and may hold a piece to the puzzle. So just decide when it feels right to share, and be proactive about asking people for recommendations, suggestions, and help.

That's a huge part of this step, asking for help and allowing yourself to be vulnerable. Admitting that you don't have it all under control and being ok with that. Remember, if you were an expert on healing, you wouldn't be in this situation. Accept what you don't know and be willing to learn at any cost.

Let Go of Control

This lesson took me a long time to learn, and I was extremely uncomfortable until I finally relinquished the need to control my experience. Like trying to plan your entire life, you can't control your journey. We honestly have very little control over anything. We can shape the direction of our lives with our thoughts, beliefs, and choices, but how it all unfolds isn't always up to us. And that's ok. It's better than ok. The universe has much bigger plans for us than we ever do.

I could never have imagined the people I'd meet and the places life would take me. Or the new information about healing and philosophies that have radically changed my beliefs and my approach to living.

If you can allow yourself to just believe that life will take care of you, you will see that there is a process happening for your benefit. Your only job is to decide what you want, to use your intuition to navigate your choices, and to get out of the way so the process can unfold naturally.

Trying to control everything will only hinder your progress. It will just slow things down and provide the opposite effect. This doesn't mean you shouldn't come up with a clear direction and decide on the next step of action to take. It just means you need to feel your way through it and stop forcing something that isn't working.

Failure Isn't Real

I'm sure you've heard this before. But in the same way that perfection will stop you in your tracks, our need to avoid failure can have the same effect. None of us want to fail. None of us want to do things poorly. But it's unrealistic to think that we can begin any new endeavor and do it right the first time, or the second, or the third. Mastery takes practice!

But this desire to get it right, or to not be seen doing it wrong, can keep us from ever starting. There is no such thing as failure. Failure is just quitting before you get to your destination. Given enough time, all of us can become accomplished at anything we set our minds to.

Does this mean anyone can become the best in the world, just because they work incredibly hard at it? Just because they set their mind to it? No. Probably not. But being the best in the world, while admirable and lofty, isn't always possible for everyone.

That doesn't mean that we shouldn't try, or that we should get discouraged. It just means that most of us are more focused on the goal than the journey. Instead of focusing on what we love, and creating more of that in our lives, we can get too focused on the outcome, and become disappointed when life doesn't turn out exactly as we've planned.

But life doesn't work that way. If you're doing what you love, does it really matter if it turns out exactly according to plan? Would life even be interesting if everything went according to a plan? I'm sure we'd feel more comfortable and secure, but also less excited.

If You Hit Resistance, Pivot

Because a health crisis can be so emotionally overwhelming, you need to stay in touch with your thoughts and feelings around everything you experience.

There were many times when situations weren't working out for me, but I was so worried that I doubted the feelings I was having. I kept placing my trust in other people's knowledge and experience over my own. Even when it didn't feel right. I mean this makes total sense right, they are the experts? The problem is, they aren't always the expert for you.

As we discussed earlier, you need to consistently tap into your intuition and the way you're feeling and trust it. Your body knows what's best for you and it's constantly giving you signals. You just need to listen. It was giving you signals before you got to this state, it still is, and it always will be. So don't dismiss your feelings around a specific person or direction. Honor them and try to get to the bottom of why you're feeling that way. If it doesn't feel right, it's time to pivot.

Pivoting means to change your angle, to change your approach. It's about hitting resistance in life, and instead of continuing to barrel into a wall, taking a step back, assessing, and making a slight turn in a different direction. This is probably one of the most common challenges I see in people – they're clear on their goals and are taking the necessary actions but aren't getting the results that they want.

This will inevitably lead to massive frustration and a lack of motivation. The key is to realize that if this is happening to you, it just means you need to modify your approach. It's a sign that you're not on the right track. This doesn't mean if you are trying to lose weight that you need to give up the entire process, it just means that you should try a different approach to reaching your goal.

Our bodies are also highly adaptive. Sometimes a certain protocol or approach works for a given amount of time and then becomes less effective. That's to be expected. Even the fittest athletes are constantly changing up their routines, because as they improve that exercise or approach becomes easier for the body. It adapts. The point is, be flexible, follow the course, and when progress seems to diminish, or doesn't feel right, be open to new angles and approaches.

BE THE NEW YOU

"Loving yourself...doesn't mean being self-absorbed or narcissistic, or disagreeing with others. Rather it means welcoming yourself as the most honored guest in your own heart, a guest worthy of respect, a loveable companion."
– MARGO ANAND

Here's where the hard work begins. It's time to start putting yourself and your healing journey first, no matter your situation. You must stop making excuses and prioritize your needs above everything else. Remember to focus on the positive aspects of your life and continually take steps in the right direction.

Put Yourself First

Now that you've begun taking some initial steps, it's imperative that you become incredibly self-interested. I dare to say, selfish. Sounds wrong doesn't it? But it really depends on the context and the details of the situation you find yourself in. Is it always bad to be selfish? To put yourself first? When you're on a healing journey and potentially fighting for your survival, don't you think it's a good time to become selfish?

You might be saying, "of course." But I see people all the time that don't know how to let go of their need to take care of others, even when it directly interferes with the goals they've established for themselves. Some of us derive so much value and pride from helping and service, that even when our lives are wildly out of balance, we still put the needs of others first.

This is not the time to take care of others. You might even be in this situation because you're amazing at taking care of others while you're consistently neglecting yourself and your needs. Helping others is incredibly important. I'm not condemning that. What I'm saying is that this process is about taking care of your needs, first and foremost. You most likely didn't set out to create a life where you could put yourself second to meet the needs of everyone else. I'm assuming you came to create, experience, and live a spectacular life filled with adventure, passion, and purpose.

Now maybe you're saying, "I have kids that depend on me, am I supposed to put them second?" The answer is, yeah, sometimes. I have an eight-year-old daughter. She's been right by my side the last few years and she's had to watch me go through some pretty difficult times. I've struggled with this a lot. Like most parents, I want to provide the best life for her. An even better childhood than I had, filled with only the best experiences. But that's not real life. When you put yourself and your needs front and center, you're teaching your children and everyone else that you matter! That your needs matter, and that your happiness matters. Think about this. What lesson would you want to pass on to your children?

- To sacrifice your health and happiness for others, because it's the right thing to do.
- To make sure you're happy and healthy first, so you can be of benefit to others.

It really hit me when I put it into that context. Even though I wasn't physically and emotionally able to be what I considered the best father over the last few years, I was teaching my daughter, with my actions and my words, about self-care and self-love. I beat myself up a lot during those times. I felt horrible for not being the fun dad and needing to lay on the couch and rest all the time. But I realized that I was doing myself a disservice by feeling so guilty. I just had to let her know that I loved her very much, but that I really needed this time to get better.

I'm sure she'll remember this period for the rest of her life. I could have tried to muster up the energy to please her, but inevitably I would have been teaching her the wrong lesson. If you aren't living your ideal life right now, at this very moment, why not? Are you putting yourself first?

Stop Making Excuses

The road to success isn't always easy. It takes incredibly focus, hard work, and consistency. One of the things I often see, is the ease with which we make excuses for why we can't achieve the goals we've set out for ourselves. A lot of the time, that's all they are, excuses. Most of us say we're too tired or don't have enough time. I get it, daily life can be overwhelming. When you try to add something else on top of your already busy routine, it just feels like too much! Especially when you're already exhausted or aren't feeling well.

The truth is, almost all of us have spare time during our day. We just choose to spend it doing things that aren't always beneficial toward reaching our goals. Watching television, spending time on the computer, playing video games, and drinking alcohol to name a few. All these activities are about decompressing and tuning out from the world. There is nothing wrong with them, but if you have the time to do any of these, you have the time to spend working toward your goals.

The issue is working toward our goals can feel exactly like that, work! Who wants to come home after a long day, make dinner, possibly put the kids to bed, and do more work? The trick is to find a way to get excited about it. When you're excited, it isn't work, it's pleasure. It's what you want to do because you believe that one day, day by day, your hard work and dedication will pay off. It's when you don't believe in yourself, or that the goal is attainable, that it becomes work.

You must get honest with yourself at this stage in the game. I understand how easy it is to use everything as an excuse. I lived in that space for a very long time. Using my health issues and the fact that I felt completely overwhelmed in every area of my life, to check out on the couch. But in all honesty, while the situation did feel extreme, I could have made different choices. I just wasn't motivated to do it. I didn't have a vision for myself, I certainly didn't have a plan, and ultimately, I didn't believe I could do it.

Challenge:

List out all the things that are stopping you from reaching your goal. Be honest with yourself. Are these real reasons? Is there anything you can do to mitigate them? Are you just self-sabotaging?

Remove Distractions

This is similar to making excuses, but it's more about making sure you're giving yourself the time and space to accomplish your goals. Even when we put ourselves first and set aside the time to create change, we can often get in our own way.

Removing distractions is about making sure you have nothing else to focus on but the task at hand. As I'm writing this chapter, I've had to shut down my email and phone. I had to put on some relaxing music, and I had to tune out the rest of world for a few hours. I'm completely used to multitasking. It's now commonplace to do multiple things at once. But we must pull ourselves away from the multitude of distractions and provide some quiet time to focus on ourselves. We need it. It's essential.

It's about creating a routine that works for you. Where you can be your most productive self. Make it into a ritual in every way that you can. You are training yourself in a new habit, and that habit should feel wholly unique. It often helps to remove yourself from your home, where distractions are everywhere.

I'm a pretty disciplined person when I set my mind to something, although I've never been able to workout at my house. Once I'm home for the day it's over, and I completely go into relaxation mode. I'm great when I set a routine that requires me to workout somewhere else, but as soon as I walk in my door, that opportunity ends. That's because over the years I've trained myself through repetition to see my home as a place to recharge, where I can leave the day behind me.

So be honest with yourself. Where are you going to be able to meet your goals? Is it at a certain place? Or a certain time of the day? Do you need to leave the house to avoid distractions? Can you set up a separate room, or area of the house to meet this goal (read, write, study, listen to audio books, meditate, exercise, etc.)?

Take it seriously, life will challenge you! Distractions are just waiting to confront you from every direction. You must be disciplined about guarding yourself against others, and yourself. There will be a hundred and one excuses why you can't stay on track, and usually only one or two reasons why you must!

Focus on the Positive

Every day we are presented with dozens of situations, each of these offer us an opportunity to choose our reaction and to learn. Unfortunately, a lot of us don't tend to react positively by nature. More often than not, we allow our minds to go to a negative place when confronted with challenging situations. Sure, it's easy to stay positive and upbeat when everything is going exactly the way you want. But how often does that happen?

Life is going to have its up and downs, and so is your journey of self-discovery and transformation. You must decide what type of person you want to be: the glass half full or the glass half empty kind? It's really that simple. We have complete control over the way we respond to any given situation. Yes, we will always have some ingrained level of emotional reaction that we may never be able to completely weed out of our system. But we don't have to be a slave to our minds or our unconscious emotional reactions.

It's our responsibility to decide how we want to react. In every moment we have a choice. Now you may not feel like you do. You may have heard some frightening news and the only thing your mind can possibly conclude is the worst outcome. But most times this just isn't the case. We often assume the worst, even when there are many possibilities that exist.

This happened to me countless times over the first year of my journey. Every imaginable thing that could possibly fall apart in my life was seemingly going wrong. I'd get so worked up about it and I was so positive that a negative outcome was going to transpire. But funny enough, in almost every single instance, things would end up working out for the best. Not necessarily in the way I had wanted, but in a way that was totally appropriate, and in nowhere near my worst fears.

You're going to have to start learning to control your mind. This is the time when you need to filter out the negative thoughts and focus solely on the positive outcome and the change you're trying to create. This means becoming the master of your thoughts. Every time a negative thought comes into your mind, you just have to let it go. It's that easy. But don't beat yourself up for it, and don't get frustrated.

Just recognize it, realize that it's not serving you, and let it go. Simultaneously, change your thoughts to something that you're excited about. Again, it's that easy. Just keep doing this throughout the day. When something comes into your mind that is distressing you, decide if it's a problem that needs to be solved, and if not, return your focus to something that brings you joy.

I want to be clear; this isn't about hiding from your problems or the reality of a serious situation. When something important needs to be dealt with, deal with it. Try your best to calm yourself, take a walk, go somewhere quiet, or just close your eyes and focus on your breath. Then make a decision from this place and just assume the best is going to happen. Assuming the worst will get you absolutely nowhere. Ever!

Remember, when challenging thoughts come into the forefront, and it's just negative chatter, redirect and focus on something that brings you joy.

Challenge:

Imagine yourself after you reach your goals. Would that person focus on the negative aspects of life? Would they get caught up in the drama and minutiae of the day to day?

Be the Change

Finally, after you've stopped making excuses, removed the distractions, and started focusing on the positive, you need to become the change. What does that mean? It means, from this day forward, you're going to act, talk, and think like the new person you want to become. It's not about pretending. It's about changing your behavior to be in alignment with what you're trying to become in your life.

It's about embodying everything we've discussed in this chapter. You're programming yourself to be a new person. You aren't going through these actions and hoping and waiting for something to happen someday. It's happening right now, and in every second! You're becoming this new version of yourself right now at this moment! You must see, think, feel, and act like the person you want to be.

That's the entire trick. It's about believing that you can do it. It's about believing that you are worthy and capable and competent. It's about deciding that on this day, that you are the change, and every action you take should be in alignment with this new version of yourself.

Real change happens gradually. But know this, if you're taking steps in the direction of your choosing, every day, you will get closer to your goal. Every healthy meal you eat, every time you exercise, every supplement you put into your body, every good night's rest you get, every book you devour, and every positive thought and conversation is one step closer!

Just imagine every one of those little choices that you make daily accumulating over time. It doesn't happen overnight. But it's happening! Constantly, consistently, and with every new positive action.

Imagine that the old you is frozen in time on the day you choose to take a new direction in your life. It no longer exists. The new version of yourself is being created every day, slowly, but surely. That's exactly what's happening. Every minute you stay on the path forward you are rewiring your brain and retraining yourself to be a different you!

If you look at anyone that's famous or that's had incredible achievements, they didn't start out that way. It took them decades to define themselves and to create incredible accomplishments or legacies. We often focus on the person as they are now and forget that they are just people, who started out simply and crafted their life through small daily choices year after year.

This is possible for all of us. You must continually focus on your goals and your vision, you can't lose sight. Our role models are no different from us. They just knew what they wanted, they believed what they wanted was possible and they never gave up!

PRACTICE PATIENCE

*"Patience is not the ability to wait, but
the ability to keep a good
attitude while waiting."*
– JOYCE MEYER

Real lasting change takes time, and this isn't a race. If you stay the course, every day you'll move closer to your goal. Remember to keep the end in sight, and to be patient.

Remember, Change Takes Time

Whatever the circumstances or situation you currently find yourself in, remember, it took you time to get here, this didn't happen overnight. Our patterns, behaviors, and beliefs develop at a young age and become rooted as we enter adulthood. You have most likely been living in this reality for a very long time. Even if it wasn't apparent. With that said, it's going to take time to create new behaviors and patterns that will ultimately create the life you want.

We are all in this for the long game. It took over two years of hard work to reclaim my health and my life, and it's not over. I will never stop working to create a better life for myself. I will never give up again! It's a daily practice, and it takes work. But if you're doing it right, it doesn't feel like work at all. It's incredibly exciting and empowering!

Looking back, everything seems so obvious now. It's similar to the way we can often look at other people's lives and see things much more clearly than they can. If we can get some distance from our situation and look at it from the outside in, it becomes clearer as well. It's our emotional attachment that can cloud our judgment. I can now see how it was all just a story in my mind, a story that kept me in that place, whether I consciously wanted to be there or not.

In all honesty, for the vast majority of those two years, it wasn't that hard. There were so many moments where I was truly enjoying myself. Does it sound impossible that when our world is falling apart, we can find joy? I can tell you, it isn't!

Of course, there were a lot of times that I was scared. Scared about my health, and scared about what was going to happen to me. Scared about the lack of control I had over my situation and scared about the unknown. But once it became clear to me that fear was just one option, that I had a choice in how I saw my circumstances, every day just continued to get better and better.

That's because I was spending an equal amount of time doing the things that I loved and that inspired me, as I was in my head worrying about everything that could possibly go wrong. Over time, as I was able to release my fear and apprehension, what was left was just a joy for life, of learning, and new experiences.

It Requires Patience

I'll be truthful. Patience is one of those things that hasn't come naturally to me. I've had to learn to slow down, to appreciate the moment, and to see the truth in this healing process. It's exactly that, a process. Like the greater process of life, you must learn to appreciate the journey, or you may never get to your desired destination.

That's the real key. You're not changing your habits and lifestyle temporarily so you can achieve a certain goal, and then just go back to the way you were. You're changing yourself, and that means changing your lifestyle, maybe in every single way imaginable. You're becoming a new version of yourself. A better, healthier, happier version. So you must find ways to enjoy this new lifestyle.

I know how difficult that can be. But what I've learned is that you have to do it your way. You have to find what works for you. You have to find activities, philosophies, and a way of living that resonate with your being. When you do, you'll become excited. You'll see what's truly possible and you will feel and know that you are on track. So be patient with yourself, and be patient with this experience. Learn to find the joy in every moment that you can. Even if you can't control the pace, you can choose your reaction!

Let Go of Your Expectations

Whatever vision you have in your mind of how this entire process is supposed to go needs to be discarded. Your journey is unique, you are unique, and your situation is unique. When you start placing expectations on how it should unfold, you are only setting yourself up for disappointment. That doesn't mean you can't have goals. It just means that if you don't hit your goal, instead of getting discouraged and wanting to throw in the towel, you just need to look for the learning. It's an opportunity to evaluate, to recalibrate, and continue forward.

There were so many times that I wanted a situation to resolve in a certain way, and it didn't. I'd have an idea in my mind of where I'd be in my healing journey at a certain time and I'd project forward what I thought was possible or realistic by a certain date. I have no idea where I came up with those expectations.

I hadn't been through this before, but somehow I had these preconceived ideas. Time and time again, I'd be let down by what I felt was a lack of progress. I assumed I'd be healed in months.

Why wasn't this happening faster? How come I felt good last week, and I feel terrible this week? Why hasn't my diet become more expansive? I've been eating this way for a year and I'm sick of it!

It's all happening exactly the way it needs to. It's all happening perfectly. The only thing that's getting in the way is you and your expectations. Allow yourself to just trust the process. Remind yourself that this *is* happening for you. It's an opportunity for you to learn, to expand your consciousness, and to change and grow. Allow it to unfold naturally, and just keep making positive, conscious decisions along the way.

If you can let go of these expectations and just trust that you are healing, that you are improving, even if it's not visible day to day, you will become the master of your journey. Know that it is happening exactly the way that it needs to, for you, in every moment.

Stop Comparing Yourself with Others

As with expectations, you must stop comparing your progress, or lack thereof, with others. Whatever lessons you need to learn, are yours to learn and in the exact way and timing that they unfold.

There are times when it's helpful to compare ourselves with others. Such as when we are taking stock of our life circumstances, or when we are creating goals for ourselves and want to use others as inspiration. But your progress, and how it unfolds, isn't really comparable to anyone else's.

There are too many factors, and it's just not important. Your belief in yourself, and in your vision for your future is all that matters.

Your Best Is Good Enough

One of the most important things to remember is to be kind to yourself. Your journey is going to have its ups and down. Some days you will feel great, and on top of the world, and other days, the complete opposite.

Try to be kind to yourself. It's just part of the process. Life is about duality. There is no light without dark, no warmth without the cold, and no joy without suffering. This duality and contrast are what amplify our appreciation for the beauty of life.

There will most likely be days when you feel unwell, unmotivated, and like a failure. Remind yourself, that this will also pass, and is only a temporary state. Allow yourself to fully experience these moments. Do not deny or push away the challenging experiences. If you allow yourself to fully embrace them, in time it will dissipate, and the energy that was holding you there will be released with it. This is part of the healing. Healing isn't just about feeling better and better every day. It's about changing, and part of changing is about releasing the old to make room for the new, and sometimes this process is uncomfortable.

I've found that if you can be kind to yourself in these moments, you can begin to see these situations as a metamorphosis. Our bodies are shedding waves of energy. The energy of the past and of our old selves, so that we can be renewed.

See these difficult times as events that you will come out of more whole and complete each time you pass through one. This isn't figuratively, this is literally. Change the way you perceive these moments. Nurture yourself through them. Take care of yourself in the way that you would take care of a child. With patience, kindness, love, and a lack of self-hatred and frustration.

This was an important lesson for me, I've been a perfectionist my entire life. My motto was, if you aren't going to do it right, then don't do it at all. I thought, why bother if it can't be the best? I worked in an industry where we made products, and I took great pride in creating something I could be proud of. But truth be told, no matter how hard I tried, no matter how many late nights I put in, nothing ever met my standards. I always wanted it to be better, and I was always disappointed that it wasn't.

This was also an issue, because I wouldn't even start a project unless I thought I could finish it, and in a way that met my standards. Can you imagine how many things I've wanted to do but never have? A lot!

I now see things very differently. I'm not saying we shouldn't strive for excellence. There is definitely a place for that in the world and in our lives. But when we are trying to change, to reclaim our lives, perfection can be the enemy. It can stop us in our tracks before we even get started. Whatever you're setting out to accomplish, sticking to the plan, taking action every day, in whatever form that takes, is perfection.

Your simple desire to change your situation, your belief that it is possible, and your small daily efforts to continue forward over weeks, months, and years, will have an incredible impact. You don't have to be the best at anything to make improvements, you just need to practice patience, and you just need to keep taking the next step!

CONCLUSION

"During your time of transformation, you might feel like everything is falling apart, but in reality, everything is coming together for your highest good. You're being pushed to evolve and get out of your comfort zone so you can live and experience your true greatness." – ANONYMOUS

I'm going to assume that at this point you've read the book and understand the concepts but may still be lacking the conviction that you need to fully reclaim your health and your life.

What I learned in this process is that your beliefs create your reality, and what you choose to believe will be the difference between failure and success in your life. That true healing is a holistic process which allows us to evaluate and recalibrate our lives to something more purposeful and meaningful.

The only request I have of you is to believe, with every cell in your body, that the path you choose is the right one for you. Whatever you decide, believing it will work will make all the difference. There is no one right solution, there is only the solution that you are dedicated to. The one that feels right to you, and the one that you put your entire heart into.

Health is a challenging topic and there are so many differing opinions. What I do know, is that if you dedicate yourself to this journey, in every way possible, that you will transform your health and your life. That all of us are capable of amazing accomplishments, but it won't happen by sitting on the sidelines. Use this crisis as an opportunity. Find a tribe, explore all your options, try new things, and find a mentor and an example to learn from. What choice do you have?

Everyone's healing journey is unique, but we all share the desire to create a better life for ourselves. One where we are healthy, where we can follow our passions, realize our dreams, and where we can spend cherished time with the people we love.

Our bodies will never lie to us. If we can get quiet, we can get clear, and then we will have access to everything we need to know about ourselves and about the world. But first, we need to take account-ability for our situations. We need to be honest that we've subconsciously created our realities and we must realize that this journey is a wake-up call. It's also an opportunity for self-discovery and self-transformation. It's filled with teachings and deep personal breakthroughs, and if you let it, it will allow you to completely transform yourself and the way you think, act, and feel.

I hope after reading this book, you're able to view the problems you've been facing in a different light. I hope you can use the framework provided to:

- Rediscover what's important to you
- See the challenges in your life as opportu-nities
- Be more empowered while facing life's oppositions
- Release fear and doubt and learn to trust yourself

- Take the next step in your process of transformation
- Reclaim your health and your life

It's time to say goodbye. I know you probably still have a lot of unanswered questions at this point in your journey. I know from experience that life isn't always easy, and sometimes it can be incredibly painful and challenging. But these experiences can teach us a lot. They taught me compassion, they taught me empathy, and they showed me another side of life that I was wholly unaware of.

I'm a stronger, more spiritually connected, and caring person than ever before. This process has also more deeply infused in me the desire to help others on their journeys.

I wish you the best! I wish you could see life the way that I do now. A life where anything is possible, if you choose to believe in yourself, and choose to just take the next step.

ACKNOWLEDGEMENTS

In my early twenties I had these recurring thoughts about writing a book about life. Of course, at that point in my own, I didn't really have a whole lot to share with the world. But for some reason this idea would keep resurfacing, and every time I would continue to dismiss it. Regardless, the concept of being an author would stay lodged in the periphery of my subconscious for the next twenty years.

Then one day, not so long ago, it hit me. My healing journey had brought me to a time and place where I had a story that I needed to tell. Writing this book is my way of documenting my experience and adding some closure to a long chapter of my life. I have no idea what's going to happen next, and I have absolutely no expectations. I just knew that this had to be done.

To the healers of the world, those who devote their lives to helping others through their mental, emotional, spiritual, and physical crisis and trauma. I want to acknowledge four of those healers, all women, who supported, guided, mentored, nurtured, and aided me on my healing journey. I doubt, with much certainty, that I would be who I am today without you.

To Maryann Schumacher, for providing me with a safe sanctuary where your coaching and breathwork training allowed me to unearth old patterns and emotions that had been holding me back from true healing. Thank you for your incredible kindness, love, and patience. You are a dear friend!

To Irene Ingalls, who introduced me to the healing power of sound. In my first session, you reawakened a part of me that had been dormant for a very long time. Thank you for taking me with you around the world on your incredible adventures, and continually opening my eyes to the mysteries of life.

To Jackie Stratton, for mending my physical body with patience and care. Your intuition and ability to listen to the body are unlike anything I've ever encountered on my twenty-year journey. You are a truly gifted healer and the world needs more people like you! I will forever be in your debt.

To Cindy Rackley, my intuitive guide and coach. Your advice and teachings have been the foundation for my recovery. You've completely changed my philosophy and beliefs and have helped me to realize my soul's true potential and purpose in this lifetime. Thank you!

ABOUT THE AUTHOR

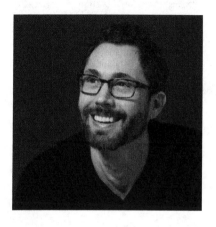

RORY REICH is a Transformational Coach, Energy Medicine Practitioner, and award-winning product Design Director. He's equally passionate about the latest scientific breakthroughs in wellness as he is about our soul's unique journey and the necessity of a holistic approach for true healing.

His mission is to help those who are out of balance achieve wholeness by learning to modify their thoughts and emotions to better align with their true desires. Throughout this process, they will begin to realize their self-impairing beliefs and discover ways of transforming them so they can create the life of their dreams. He lives in Seattle, Washington, with his daughter, Sophia.

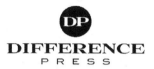

ABOUT
DIFFERENCE PRESS

Difference Press is the exclusive publishing arm of The Author Incubator, an educational company for entrepreneurs – including life coaches, healers, consultants, and community leaders – looking for a comprehensive solution to get their books written, published, and promoted. Its founder, Dr. Angela Lauria, has been bringing to life the literary ventures of hundreds of authors-in-transformation since 1994.

A boutique-style self-publishing service for clients of The Author Incubator, Difference Press boasts a fair and easy-to-understand profit structure, low-priced author copies, and author-friendly contract terms. Most importantly, all of our #incubatedauthors maintain ownership of their copyright at all times.

Let's Start a Movement with Your Message

In a market where hundreds of thousands of books are published every year and are never heard from again, The Author Incubator is different. Not only do all Difference Press books reach Amazon bestseller status, but all of our authors are actively changing lives and making a difference.

Since launching in 2013, we've served over 500 authors who came to us with an idea for a book and were able to write it and get it self-published in less than 6 months. In addition, more than 100 of those books were picked up by traditional publishers and are now available in book stores. We do this by selecting the highest quality and highest potential applicants for our future programs.

Our program doesn't only teach you how to write a book – our team of coaches, developmental editors, copy editors, art directors, and marketing experts incubate you from having a book idea to being a published, bestselling author, ensuring that the book you create can actually make a difference in the world. Then we give you the training you need to use your book to make the difference in the world, or to create a business out of serving your readers.

Are You Ready to Make a Difference?

You've seen other people make a difference with a book. Now it's your turn. If you are ready to stop watching and start taking massive action, go to **http://theauthorincubator.com/apply/.**

"Yes, I'm ready!"

OTHER BOOKS BY DIFFERENCE PRESS

Reverse Button™: Learn What the Doctors Aren't Telling You, Avoid Back Surgery, and Get Your Full Life Back by Abby Beauchamp

Never Too Late for Love: The Successful Woman's Guide to Online Dating in the Second Half of Life by Joan Bragar, EdD

Stronger Together: My MS Story by Chloe Cohen

Yogini's Dilemma: To Be, or Not to Be, a Yoga Teacher? by Nicole A. Grant

Come Alive: Find Your Passion, Change Your Life, Change the World! by Jodi Hadsell

Meant For More: Stop Secretly Struggling and Become a Force to Be Reckoned With by Mia Hewett

Lord, Please Save My Marriage: A Christian Woman's Guide to Thrive, Despite Her Husband's Drunken Rants by Christine Lennard

If I'm so Zen, Why Is My Hair Falling Out?: How Past Trauma and Anxiety Manifest in the Physical Body by Amanda Lera

Heal Your Trauma, Heal Your Marriage: 7 Steps to Root, Rebound, and Rise by Dr. Cheri L. McDonald

WELCOME to the Next Level: 3 Secrets to Become Unstuck, Take Action, and Rise Higher in Your Career by Sonya L. Sigler

Embrace Your Psychic Gifts: The Guide to Spiritual Awakening by Deborah Sudarsky

Leverage: The Guide to End Your Binge Eating by Linda Vang

Under the Sleeve: Find Help for Your Child Who Is Cutting by Dr. Stacey Winters

THANK YOU

Thank you so much for reading *Transform Yourself Through Disease*. If you've made it this far, I know you are more ready than ever to reclaim your health and your life. I truly understand how challenging this process can be, and I want to help and support you as much as possible. I would love to hear more about your healing journey and your successes.

Please keep in touch with me on Facebook and Instagram. You can share your learnings by tagging me and using **#transformyourselfthroughdisease**, or visit me at **RoryReich.com** for more resources. You can always drop me an email if that's easier at **info@RoryReich.com**.

Thanks,
Rory Reich